MW00960857

Fructose-Free Living

A Cookbook for Intolerance-Friendly Meals

Eloke

© [2024], Eloke.

All rights reserved. This book, or any portion thereof, may not be reproduced or used in any manner whatsoever without the express written permission of the author, except for the use of brief quotations in a book review or scholarly journal.

For inquiries regarding permissions, contact:

[stellaeloke6@gmail.com]

Eloke

Introduction

Welcome to "Fructose-Free Living: A Cookbook for Intolerance-Friendly Meals." If you've picked up this book, you might be one of many people dealing with the intricacies of fructose intolerance. Whether you are newly diagnosed, have been dealing with symptoms for years, or are looking for delicious recipes that will not jeopardize your health, you have arrived to the correct spot.

Understanding Fructose intolerance

Fructose intolerance, also known as fructose malabsorption, is when the body has trouble digesting fructose, a sugar found in many fruits, sweets, and processed meals. This illness can cause a variety of unpleasant symptoms, including bloating, gas, abdominal pain, and diarrhea. For many people, these symptoms can be both physically painful and socially isolating. Imagine attending a gathering and being unable to participate in the joy of shared meals—this is a reality for those who are fructose intolerant.

While the specifics of fructose intolerance vary from person to person, understanding the basic mechanics might give you confidence. The small intestine struggles to absorb fructose effectively, so it travels to the colon and ferments. This fermentation process causes gas and discomfort, making many people concerned about what they can safely eat.

The good news is that many people find that following a fructose-free diet helps them feel much better. You may find yourself enjoying meals without the burden of discomfort or humiliation. The goal is to learn which foods to avoid and to seek out alternative ingredients that are both safe and satisfying.

The Importance of A Fructose-Free Diet

Starting a fructose-free diet may appear overwhelming at first. After all, the world of food is full of flavors, sensations, and experiences, many of which come from fructose-rich fruits and sweeteners. However, eliminating fructose from your diet can have a dramatic effect.

A fructose-free diet is more than just what you can't eat; it's about embracing the wide range of options accessible to you. Many people report feeling better overall after cutting out sugar. Benefits of this dietary adjustment include improved digestion, reduced bloating, and enhanced energy levels. Furthermore, by focusing on complete, unprocessed meals, you may unintentionally adopt a healthier overall lifestyle.

This diet is important for more than just your physical wellness. Emotional well-being is an important consideration. Living with food intolerances can cause anxiety and stress. However, by mastering a fructose-free diet, you may reclaim control of your eating habits, enhance your confidence, and build a positive relationship with food.

This voyage might also provide opportunities for culinary innovation. Cooking and experimenting with new ingredients may be really satisfying. As you experiment with various flavors and meals, you may find latent culinary talents or perhaps rediscover your passion for cooking.

How To Use This Cookbook

This cookbook is intended to be your companion on your road to a fructose-free diet. Each recipe has been painstakingly created to ensure that it is not only safe for persons with fructose intolerance, but also delicious and fulfilling for everyone at the table. Whether you're cooking for yourself, family, or friends, these recipes will dazzle.

Organize Your Kitchen

Before you begin the recipes, take a moment to arrange your kitchen. Remove any high-fructose foods that may cause pain, and refill your cupboard with fructose-free options. The first chapter will walk you through the necessary pantry essentials and equipment to make cooking pleasurable and efficient.

Exploring Recipes

As you progress through the chapters, you will discover a wide range of recipes, from breakfast to dessert. Each part is designed to provide a balanced assortment of meals that may be easily integrated into your regular routine.

Breakfast Ideas: Get your day started right with stimulating breakfast alternatives like smoothies, savory egg dishes, and sweet sweets that are all fructose-free.

Lunch Recipes: Choose from a variety of salads and substantial soups to keep you fuelled and focused throughout the day.

Dinner Delights: Gather around the table for tasty dinner recipes, featuring meat, seafood, and vegetarian alternatives that are sure to please a crowd.

Snacks and Appetizers: Discover quick and nutritious snacks to satisfy cravings and share with family and friends.

Desserts: You can indulge your sweet craving without stress. With recipes for cakes, cookies, and frozen sweets, you may indulge in dessert guilt-free.

Meal Plans: To help you transition to a fructose-free lifestyle, we've included a one-week meal plan with grocery lists. This practical method will assist you in navigating the problems of meal preparation while also ensuring that you have a diverse selection of meals to enjoy.

Practical Tips

Throughout the book, you will find recommendations on how to modify recipes to your liking, storage suggestions for leftovers, and guidance on dining out safely. Whether you're at home or on the go, this cookbook will give you the information and confidence you need to succeed in a fructose-free environment.

Community & Support

Finally, realize that you are not alone on this path. Many people share your experiences, and engaging with support groups or online forums can be really beneficial. This cookbook will serve as the starting point for your journey, providing not only recipes but also a sense of community as you learn to manage the obstacles of fructose intolerance together.

Eloke

Chapter One: Kitchen Essentials.

Beginning a fructose-free journey necessitates not only a dietary shift, but also a careful attitude to your kitchen. In this chapter, we'll go over the basics of stocking your pantry with fructose-free goods, the necessary cooking equipment, and meal prep methods to make your cooking experience more fun and efficient. With the correct tools and materials, you can easily prepare tasty meals that suit your lifestyle while also satisfying your taste buds.

Fructose-free pantry staples.

When adjusting to a fructose-free diet, your pantry is your first line of defense. Stocking it with the correct ingredients is critical for ensuring you have everything you need to prepare meals that are both delicious and safe. Here's a list of crucial fructose-free pantry items.

1. Grains and Cereals

Choose whole grains and cereals that are low in fructose. Some great options include:

Rice: White, brown, jasmine, and basmati rice are all good choices.

Oats: Both rolled and steel-cut oats are healthful and flexible. Use them for breakfast or in baked dishes.

Quinoa: This protein-rich grain is ideal for salads and sides.

Cornmeal and polenta are both good base ingredients for many meals.

2. Legumes and pulses

Beans and lentils are excellent sources of protein and fiber. Consider options such as:

Black beans have a rich flavor and are ideal for soups and salads.

Chickpeas are great for creating hummus and adding to salads.

Lentils are versatile and cook quickly, making them ideal for soups, stews, and salads.

3. Proteins

Protein sources are essential for a nutritious diet. Here is what to include:

Meats include fresh cuts of beef, chicken, turkey, and pork. Avoid processed meats that can include high-fructose components.

Fish and seafood: Fresh or frozen fish, shrimp, and scallops are excellent protein sources.

Eggs are a versatile item for breakfast, salads, and baking.

Tofu and Tempeh are excellent vegetarian protein sources that are low in sugar.

4. Dairy and alternatives

Choose dairy products that are devoid of fructose. Here are some options:

Milk can be whole, low fat, or lactose-free.

Yogurt: Plain or Greek yogurt with no additional sweeteners.

Cheese: Most hard cheeses are safe, but soft cheeses should be tested for added sugar.

If you prefer non-dairy alternatives, consider:

Check the labels of almond milk to be sure there are no added sugars.

Coconut Milk is an excellent choice for cooking and smoothies.

5. Oils and Vinegar

Cooking oils and vinegars can enhance flavors without adding sugar. Recommended alternatives include:

Olive oil is a mainstay in cooking and salads.

Coconut Oil: Ideal for baking and frying.

Vinegars include balsamic, apple cider, and red wine vinegar (check for added sweeteners).

6. Sweeteners

Finding fructose-free sweeteners is critical for baking and cooking. Consider the following options:

Stevia is a natural, calorie-free sweetener.

Erythritol is a sugar alcohol that delivers sweetness without calories.

Monk Fruit: Another natural sweetener that has no fructose.

7. Spices & herbs

Fresh or dried herbs and spices enhance flavor without including fructose. Stock up:

Basil, oregano, and thyme: ideal for Mediterranean meals.

Cinnamon and nutmeg are excellent for imparting warmth to baked products.

Garlic and onion are essential for enhancing flavor in savory recipes.

8. Canned and jarred goods

Having a few canned and jarred foods on hand can help you prepare meals faster. Choose:

Canned tomatoes are ideal for sauces and stews.

Canned coconut milk is ideal for curries and desserts.

Nut butters: Almond or peanut butter with no additional sugar.

9. Snacks

Finding snacks that fit into a fructose-free diet can be difficult, but there are plenty of possibilities.

Rice cakes are light and adaptable, and they pair well with spreads.

Popcorn: Air-popped with no additional flavoring.

Nuts and seeds: Almonds, walnuts, and pumpkin seeds are all excellent snacks.

10. Baking Supplies

You can still enjoy baked goods without fructose. Store your baking ingredients with:

Gluten-Free Flour: Almond and coconut flour can be used in a variety of recipes.

Baking soda and powder are essential for leavening baked goods.

Unsweetened Cocoa Powder: Perfect for chocolate treats.

Essential Cooking Equipment

Equipping your kitchen with the necessary tools can greatly improve your cooking experience. Here's a list of necessary kitchen tools that will make creating fructose-free meals easier and more enjoyable:

1. Knives

A decent knife set is a must-have in every kitchen. A chef's knife, paring knife, and serrated knife will meet the majority of your slicing, chopping, and dicing requirements.

2. Cutting Boards

Having multiple cutting boards is beneficial, particularly for preventing cross-contamination. Use one for meat and the other for fruits and veggies.

3. Measuring cup and spoon

Precision is essential in cooking and baking. A set of measuring cups and spoons ensures that you take the correct measurements every time.

4. Mixing Bowls

A range of mixing bowls of varying sizes will allow you to efficiently prepare ingredients and combine batters. Look for dishes with lids for convenient storing.

5. Pots and pans.

A decent set of pots and pans is crucial for cooking. Invest in:

Non-stick skillets are ideal for frying eggs and sautéing veggies.

Sauce pans are ideal for sauces, cereals, and soups.

Stock Pot: Ideal for preparing huge quantities of soup or pasta.

6. Baking sheet and pans

To bake, you will need a few essentials:

Baking sheets are ideal baking cookies and roasting veggies.

Loaf Pan: Ideal for fast breads and meatloafs.

Muffin Tin: Perfect for cupcakes and portioned breakfast items.

7. Food Processor

A food processor can help you save time and effort when chopping, combining, or pureeing ingredients. Look for one with a variety of attachments for maximum adaptability.

8. Blender

A high-speed blender is required for making smoothies, soups, and sauces. It is also useful for making nut butters and puréeing fruits and vegetables.

9. Slow Cooker or Instant Pot?

These equipment are ideal for hands-free cooking. A slow cooker can help you make stews and soups, whereas an Instant Pot can shorten cooking times for cereals and meats.

10. Utensils

Using the proper utensils can make cooking more enjoyable. Stock your kitchen with the following:

Spatulas: Silicone spatulas are ideal for mixing and scraping.

Whisks are essential for mixing batters and sauces.

Tongs are ideal for turning meats and presenting salads.

11. Storage containers

Invest in a set of high-quality storage containers for leftovers. Glass containers with airtight lids are great for keeping food and may be used in the microwave or oven.

Meal Planning Tips for Fructose-Free Cooking

Meal planning is a game changer for anyone following a fructose-free diet. It saves time while also ensuring that you always have healthful, safe meals on hand. Here are some meal prep suggestions that will help you succeed.

1. Plan your meals.

Begin each week by organizing your meals. Choose meals from this cookbook that appeal to you while maintaining a healthy balance of protein, grains, and veggies. Planning ahead of time helps to reduce stress and makes shopping easier.

2. Create a shopping list.

Create a thorough grocery list based on your food plan. Stick to your list to prevent making spontaneous purchases of high-fructose items.

3. Batch cooking.

Set aside a few hours per week to batch cook. Prepare huge quantities of grains, proteins, and veggies for use during the week. For example, prepare a large batch of quinoa or roast a tray of vegetables to use in various meals.

4. Pre-Chopped Vegetables

Chopping vegetables can be time-consuming. Take the time to cut veggies and store them in sealed containers for convenient access throughout the week. This makes it easy to prepare salads, stir fries, and side dishes.

5. Portioning Meals

After cooking, divide your meals into individual portions. This will make it easier to grab a meal when you don't have much time. Consider utilizing translucent containers so you can see what's accessible.

6. Utilize Freezing.

Freezing is a great strategy to extend the shelf life of your food. Soups, stews, and baked dishes can be frozen and then reheated later. Label and date your containers for easy identification.

7. Keep snacks on hand.

Make healthful snacks in advance. Portion nuts, cut up fruits and veggies, or prepare energy balls for quick snacks throughout the week.

8. Stay organized.

Keep your kitchen organized so that you can readily locate materials and tools. An organized kitchen may make cooking more fun and efficient.

9. Experiment and adapt.

As you gain confidence in cooking with fructose-free ingredients, don't be afraid to experiment with flavors and textures. Your palette will evolve, and you will discover new favorite combinations that will add excitement to your meals.

Transitioning to a fructose-free lifestyle can seem difficult at first, but by stocking your kitchen with the necessary items, you can make the process easier. This chapter has created the framework for your journey, teaching you the value of stocking a fructose-free pantry, accumulating necessary cooking tools, and using meal prep techniques to make your life easier. As you continue to explore the delectable possibilities of a fructose-free diet, remember that the kitchen is your canvas, and with the correct tools and ingredients, you can create culinary masterpieces that nourish your body while satisfying your cravings.

Let's go together into the world of delectable and safe meals that complement your lifestyle!

Chapter 2: Breakfast Ideas.

Breakfast is frequently regarded as the most essential meal of the day, and with good reason. It's the fuel that jumpstarts your metabolism and sets the tone for the day. If you avoid fructose, you may be concerned that your breakfast selections are limited. However, a universe of tasty and fulfilling options awaits you! This chapter will look at a range of breakfast alternatives that are not only simple to prepare but also packed with taste and nutrition. Let's learn how to make your mornings more enjoyable with smoothies, breakfast bowls, savory omelets, and sweet desserts.

Smoothies & juices

Energizing Smoothies

Smoothies are an excellent way to incorporate nutritious value into your daily routine. They're simple to make, easily adaptable, and can bring a welcome start to your day. When making smoothies, make sure you use fructose-free products. Here are some advice and recipe ideas to help you get started:

Base Ingredients:

Unsweetened Almond Milk: A great low-calorie substitute for dairy, almond milk is easy on the stomach and high in nutrients. You can also experiment with different milk replacements, such as coconut or oat milk, as long as they have no added sugars.

Spinach or Kale: Leafy greens are high in nutrients and fiber, yet they contain no sugar. They combine easily and are almost flavorless in smoothies, making them ideal for delivering a nutritious boost.

Greek yogurt is a great source of protein and adds creaminess to smoothies. Choose basic, unsweetened types to keep your smoothie fructose-free.

Flavor Enhancers.

Avocado: In addition to its velvety texture, avocado is high in healthy fats, which keep you fuller for longer.

Frozen Berries: While some fruits are high in fructose, berries such as strawberries, blueberries, and raspberries are often lower in sugar and can be had in moderation. They offer a beautiful color and flavor without being overly sweet.

Chia seeds, flaxseeds, and walnuts can be blended in to provide additional nutrients and healthy fats.

Recipe idea: Green Power Smoothie

1 cup of unsweetened almond milk.

1 cup of fresh spinach.

½ ripe avocado.

Eloke

½ cup frozen blueberries.

1 tablespoon of chia seeds.

Blend till smooth, then enjoy the refreshing green power!

Refreshing juices

Juices are also an excellent breakfast alternative, providing a refreshing start to the day. When producing juices, use low-fructose vegetables and fruits. Here are a few excellent combinations:

Cucumber and Mint Juice

Cucumber is hydrating and low in calories, so it makes an excellent base for a refreshing drink. Combine it with fresh mint for an energizing morning beverage.

One medium cucumber, peeled and cut

A handful of fresh mint leaves.

Juice from 1 lemon

Water as needed.

Blend and pass through a fine sieve.

Carrot and Ginger Juice

Carrots are sweet but low in fructose, and ginger provides a spicy bite that helps aid digestion.

Two medium carrots, chopped.

1 inch of fresh ginger, peeled

1 cup water.

Blend and strain to create a zesty juice!

Breakfast Bowls

Breakfast bowls have taken the culinary world by storm, and for good reason: they are versatile and can be made with a variety of ingredients to suit your taste and dietary requirements. Here are some ideas for making delicious fructose-free breakfast bowls.

Quinoa Breakfast Bowl

Quinoa is a protein-rich grain that makes a terrific base for breakfast bowls. It's gluten-free and adaptable, making it a great option for a hearty breakfast.

Recipe idea: Quinoa Bowl with Nuts and Seeds

1 cup cooked quinoa.

1/2 cup unsweetened almond milk.

1 tablespoon almond butter.

2 tablespoons mixed nuts (almonds, walnuts)

One tablespoon pumpkin seeds.

Sprinkle with cinnamon.

Combine all of the ingredients in a bowl and enjoy a protein-rich breakfast with healthy fats.

Chia Seed Pudding.

Chia seeds are high in omega-3 fatty acids and fiber, and they may be made into a delicious creamy pudding for breakfast.

Recipe Idea: Coconut Chia Pudding.

¼ cup Chia seeds

1 cup coconut milk, unsweetened

1 teaspoon of vanilla extract.

A sprinkle of cinnamon.

Fresh berries for topping.

In a bowl, combine chia seeds, coconut milk, vanilla essence, and cinnamon. Stir thoroughly and refrigerate overnight. In the morning, top with fresh berries for a delicious start to the day.

Savory Options: Omelets and Scrambles.

If you want a more substantial breakfast, savory options such as omelets and scrambles can be extremely fulfilling. They are quick to make and may be stuffed with a variety of vegetables and proteins.

Vegetable-Packed Omelet

Eggs are an excellent source of protein, and when coupled with nutrient-dense vegetables, they form a tasty and full meal.

Recipe Idea: Spinach and Feta Omelet

Two huge eggs.

A handful of fresh spinach.

¼ cup crumbled feta cheese

Add salt and pepper to taste.

Cook in a nonstick skillet until done.

This omelet is not only tasty, but also high in nutrients, keeping you energized throughout the morning.

Scrambled Eggs with Avocado

Avocado is an excellent compliment to eggs, giving smoothness and healthful fats. This combo is ideal for a simple but filling breakfast.

Recipe Idea: Avocado Scramble

Two huge eggs.

1/2 ripe avocado, chopped.

Add salt and pepper to taste.

Cook the eggs in a skillet, then add the diced avocado just before serving.

This dish is quick to prepare and will keep you satisfied until noon.

Sweet treats include muffins and pancakes.

Just because you are avoiding fructose does not mean you can't enjoy delicious breakfast goodies! With a little imagination, you can make muffins and pancakes that are both tasty and healthy.

Flourless Banana Muffins

When it comes to limiting your fructose intake, bananas can be consumed in moderation. These flourless muffins are moist and tasty.

Recipe: Flourless Banana Muffins

Two ripe bananas.

Two huge eggs.

1/2 cup almond butter.

1 teaspoon of baking powder.

Combine all ingredients and bake at 350°F (175°C) for 15-20 minutes.

These muffins are ideal for a quick breakfast on the run.

Oatmeal pancakes.

Oatmeal makes an excellent pancake basis, providing fiber and nutrients without adding sugar.

Recipe Ideas: Oatmeal Pancakes

1 cup rolled oats.

1 cup almond milk.

One huge egg.

1 teaspoon of baking powder.

Combine all ingredients and fry in a nonstick skillet until golden brown on both sides.

Serve with a sprinkle of pure maple syrup (in moderation) or a dollop of yogurt for a delicious breakfast.

Even if you avoid fructose, breakfast may be a delicious and healthful way to start the day. The recipes and ideas offered in this chapter are intended to encourage creativity and make mornings more delightful. From refreshing smoothies and hearty breakfast bowls to spicy omelets and sweet sweets, you can discover a variety of flavors and textures to suit your dietary requirements.

As you try these breakfast alternatives, keep in mind that your palate will change over time. Accept the opportunity to test new ingredients and combinations that will tantalize your taste senses while feeding your body. With so many tasty alternatives available, breakfast can quickly become one of your favorite meals of the day!

Chapter 3: Lunch Recipes.

Lunch is more than simply a meal; it's a chance to recharge and re-energize yourself for the day. When eating fructose-free, it's easy to fall into the trap of monotonous meals, but this chapter will present you with vivid, fulfilling, and nutritious lunch recipes that can be prepared quickly and enjoyed by everyone. From fresh salads and homemade dressings to hearty soups and wraps, let's explore the world of delectable lunch choices that are ideal for your fructose-free diet.

Salad and Dressing

Salads can be the focal point of a delicious lunch, providing a range of textures and flavors while being quite easy to modify. Whether you favor crisp greens, hearty grains, or vivid vegetables, there is a salad for you.

Colorful grain salads

Grain salads are an excellent way to include healthful ingredients in your meal. They give a satisfying foundation while allowing for an infinite number of vegetable and protein combinations.

Recipe Idea: Quinoa and Chickpea Salad

Ingredients:

1 cup cooked quinoa.

1 cup canned chickpeas, drained and rinsed.

1 cup of diced cucumbers.

1 cup halved cherry tomatoes.

¼ cup chopped fresh parsley.

1/4 cup olive oil.

2 teaspoons of lemon juice.

Add salt and pepper to taste.

Instructions:

In a large mixing basin, combine the quinoa, chickpeas, cucumbers, tomatoes, and parsley.

In a separate small bowl, combine olive oil, lemon juice, salt, and pepper.

Toss the salad with the dressing until well combined. Allow it to sit for at least 10 minutes to let the flavors blend.

This salad is not only colorful and visually appealing, but it also has plenty of protein and fiber to keep you satisfied until supper.

Crisp green salads

A fresh green salad is a staple lunchtime option that may be endlessly customized. Combining different greens, vegetables, and proteins can result in a delicious combination that you'll look forward to each day.

Recipe Idea: Spinach and Avocado Salad

Ingredients:

4 cups of fresh spinach.

One ripe avocado, chopped

1/2 cup sliced radishes.

1/2 cup shredded carrots.

¼ cup pumpkin seeds

2 tablespoons olive oil.

1 tablespoon of balsamic vinegar.

Add salt and pepper to taste.

Instructions:

In a large salad bowl, mix together the spinach, avocado, radishes, carrots, and pumpkin seeds.

In a small bowl, combine olive oil, balsamic vinegar, salt, and pepper.

Drizzle the dressing over the salad right before serving and gently mix to blend.

The creamy avocado pairs well with the crisp radishes and seeds, creating a delicious contrast of flavors and textures.

Homemade dressings

Store-bought dressings frequently include hidden sugars, including fructose. Making your own dressings at home gives you control over the ingredients and ensures they meet your dietary restrictions.

Recipe Idea: Lemon Tahini Dressing

Ingredients:

¼ cup tahini

Juice from 1 lemon

1 clove garlic, minced

Water to thin (as needed).

Add salt and pepper to taste.

Instructions:

In a bowl, combine the tahini, lemon juice, and garlic.

Add water gradually until the required consistency is achieved.

Season with salt and pepper.

This creamy dressing can be drizzled over salads, served as a dip, or spread on sandwiches for extra taste.

Sandwiches and Wraps

Sandwiches and wraps are quite adaptable and may be filled with a wide range of ingredients to suit your preferences. The perfect combination may elevate a basic meal to something intriguing and satisfying.

Delightful Wraps

Wraps are ideal for on-the-go lunches. They can be filled with a variety of ingredients, providing for flexibility and customisation.

Recipe Idea: Turkey and Spinach Wrap.

Ingredients:

One large whole wheat or gluten-free wrap.

4 slices of turkey breast (look for added sweeteners)

1 cup of fresh spinach.

1/2 cup shredded carrots.

¼ avocado, sliced

Mustard or hummus to spread

Instructions:

Spread mustard or hummus on the wrap.

Layer the turkey with spinach, carrots, and avocado.

Roll firmly and cut in half.

This wrap is healthful, easy to prepare, and ideal for lunch at home or on the go.

Classic Sandwiches

A classic sandwich has a certain cozy quality. You may improve your lunch game by using fresh ingredients that are both delicious and fructose free.

Recipe Idea: Grilled Chicken Sandwich

Ingredients:

2 slices of whole-grain bread (look for fructose-free alternatives)

One grilled chicken breast, sliced

1/2 cup arugula or spinach.

¼ cup sliced tomato

2 tablespoons of pesto (preferably homemade)

Instructions:

Toast the bread till golden brown.

Spread pesto on one side of each slice.

Place the chicken, arugula, and tomatoes on one slice, then top with the other.

This grilled chicken sandwich is flavorful and fulfilling, making it ideal for any lunch hour.

Hearty soups

Soups are a great lunch option, especially when they're substantial and nutritious. They are frequently simple to make ahead of time and can be saved for fast lunches throughout the week.

Wholesome Vegetable Soup

A vegetable soup is not only warming, but it also makes good use of any leftover vegetables you may have.

Recipe Idea: Hearty Vegetable Soup

Ingredients:

1 tablespoon of olive oil.

One onion, chopped

2 garlic cloves, minced

Two carrots, sliced

Two celery stalks, cut

One zucchini, diced

1 can of diced tomatoes (check for extra sugar)

4 cups veggie broth.

1 teaspoon of dried oregano.

Add salt and pepper to taste.

Instructions:

In a large pot, heat the olive oil over medium heat. Cook the onion and garlic until softened.

Cook the carrots and celery for 5 minutes.

Stir in the zucchini, tomatoes, broth, oregano, salt, and pepper. Bring to a boil, then reduce the heat and simmer for 30 minutes.

This soup is rich and filling, ideal for a cold day or when you need a warm lunch.

Creamy Potato Soup

Potato soup may be rich and luscious while remaining fructose-free. It's a lovely alternative that can be prepared in huge quantities.

Recipe Idea: Creamy Potato Soup

Ingredients:

4 medium potatoes, peeled and chopped

1 onion, chopped

2 cups veggie broth.

1 cup of unsweetened almond milk.

Add salt and pepper to taste.

Instructions:

In a pot, combine the potatoes, onion, and vegetable broth. Bring to a boil, then cook until the potatoes are cooked.

Blend the soup till smooth, then stir in the almond milk. Season with salt and pepper.

This creamy potato soup is both cozy and filling, making it ideal for lunch any day of the week.

Quick and Easy Rice Dishes

Rice dishes are a quick and filling lunch choice that may be made in a variety of ways. They are adaptable, allowing you to mix and match components depending on what you have on hand.

Fried Rice

Fried rice is a popular dish that may be personalized with your preferred vegetables and proteins. It's an excellent way to repurpose leftover rice and make a hearty supper.

Recipe Idea: Vegetable Fried Rice

Ingredients:

Eloke

2 cups of cooked brown rice.

1 tablespoon of sesame oil.

1 cup mixed veggies, such as carrots, peas, and bell peppers.

Two eggs, beaten

Soy sauce (look for low sodium alternatives)

Instructions:

Heat the sesame oil in a large skillet over medium heat. Add the mixed vegetables and cook until tender.

Push the vegetables to one side while scrambling the eggs in the pan.

Once the eggs are cooked, mix in the prepared rice and soy sauce. Stir everything together and simmer until thoroughly cooked.

This vegetable fried rice is bright, nutritious, and ideal for a quick lunch.

Rice Bowl

Rice bowls are another great alternative, as they allow for a range of toppings and flavors.

Recipe Idea: Chicken and Broccoli Rice Bowl

Ingredients:

2 cups of cooked brown rice.

One grilled chicken breast, sliced

1 cup steaming broccoli.

¼ cup teriyaki sauce (look for fructose-free alternatives)

Instructions:

In a bowl, combine cooked rice, cut chicken, and steamed broccoli.

Drizzle with teriyaki sauce and enjoy!

Eloke

This rice dish is full, tasty, and ideal for a busy day.

Lunch does not have to be dull or limiting if you live a fructose-free diet. With the recipes and ideas in this chapter, you may prepare a range of delectable and fulfilling meals that will keep you energized throughout the day. From fresh salads and substantial soups to inventive wraps and quick rice meals, there's something for everyone to enjoy.

Thank You for Reading!

I want to take a moment to personally thank you for choosing to read fructose- free living. Your time and effort are sincerely appreciated, and I hope this book has provided you with significant ideas and skills for success.

As I continue to grow as an author, your feedback is immensely essential to me. I would love to hear your thoughts—whether positive or constructive—so I can grow and make future works even more helpful and fascinating.

If you found this book beneficial or if there's something you feel could be enhanced, I respectfully ask that you provide an honest review. Your insights will not only help me improve but also assist other readers in locating the correct information.

Eloke

Thank you again for your support, and I look forward to hearing from you!

Warm regards,

Chapter 4: Dinner Delights.

Dinner is frequently the highlight of the day, providing an opportunity to unwind and share a nice meal with family and friends. Dinner can be colorful and tasty even if you follow a fructose-free diet. This chapter includes a variety of enticing dishes for poultry, meat, fish, vegetarian, and vegan alternatives, as well as tasty stir-fries. Each recipe is intended to be delicious, nutritious, and easy to prepare, guaranteeing that your dinner table is full of delectable meals.

Poultry and Meat dishes

Poultry and meat can be the highlight of your dinner menu, with rich flavors and pleasant textures. These recipes are not only simple to prepare, but also provide a full supper without extra sugar.

Herb-Roasted Chicken

Classic herb-roasted chicken is ideal for family gatherings or a quick weekday dinner. The herb blend produces a savory aroma that fills your kitchen.

Recipe idea: Herb-Roasted Chicken

Ingredients:

1 entire chicken (about 4 pounds)

3 tablespoons olive oil.

2 teaspoons of fresh rosemary, chopped

2 tablespoons fresh thyme, chopped.

4 garlic cloves, minced

Add salt and pepper to taste.

Lemon wedges for serving.

Instructions:

Preheat the oven to 375°F (190° C).

Pat the chicken dry and put it in a roasting pan.

In a small bowl, combine olive oil, rosemary, thyme, garlic, salt, and pepper.

Rub the herb mixture all over the chicken, even beneath the skin, for more flavor.

Roast for approximately 1 hour and 15 minutes, or until the internal temperature reaches 165°F (75°C).

Allow it to rest for ten minutes before carving. Serve with lemon wedges.

This dish is not only simple to make, but it produces juicy, flavorful meat that works well with roasted vegetables or a fresh salad.

Beef Stir-fry

Stir-fries are a quick and delectable method to prepare dinner, allowing you to combine different vegetables and proteins.

Recipe Idea: Beef Stir-Fry

Ingredients:

1 pound beef sirloin, cut thin

2 tablespoons soy sauce (make sure it is fructose-free)

1 tablespoon of cornstarch.

2 tablespoons of vegetable oil.

2 cups assorted bell peppers, sliced

1 cup of broccoli florets.

2 garlic cloves, minced

1 inch of grated ginger.

Cooked brown rice for dishing.

Instructions:

In a bowl, combine the beef, soy sauce, and cornstarch. Allow to marinate for 15 minutes.

Heat 1 tablespoon oil in a large skillet over medium-high heat. Add the steak and cook until browned. Remove and set aside.

In the same skillet, combine the remaining oil, bell peppers, broccoli, garlic, and ginger. Stir-fry for about 5 minutes, until the vegetables are soft and crisp.

Return the beef to the skillet and stir until combined. Serve with cooked brown rice.

This beef stir-fry is not only tasty, but it can also be customized by adding any of your favorite vegetables!

Seafood Options:

Seafood has a wide range of flavors and nutritional advantages, making it an excellent choice for dinner. Whether you favor fish or shellfish, these recipes will suit any taste.

Lemon Garlic Butter Shrimp.

Shrimp cooks quickly and is ideal for a light yet classy dinner. This recipe combines the tastes of garlic and lemon to create a dinner that will impress.

Recipe idea: Lemon Garlic Butter Shrimp

Ingredients:

1 pound of big shrimp, peeled and deveined

3 tablespoons butter.

4 garlic cloves, minced

Juice from 1 lemon

Zest from 1 lemon

Add salt and pepper to taste.

Fresh parsley for garnish.

In a large skillet, melt the butter over medium heat. Sauté garlic until aromatic, about 1 minute.

Add the shrimp to the skillet and cook for 2-3 minutes per side, or until pink and opaque.

Stir in the lemon juice, zest, salt, and pepper. Toss to coat the shrimp with the sauce.

Serve immediately and garnish with fresh parsley.

This shrimp dish is ideal served with steamed asparagus or over quinoa for a complete dinner.

Baked Salmon and Dill

Baking salmon is a simple method to prepare this healthful fish while keeping it moist and tasty.

Recipe Idea: Baked Salmon with Dill

Eloke

Ingredients:

4 Salmon fillets

2 tablespoons olive oil.

2 teaspoons of fresh dill, chopped

Juice from 1 lemon

Add salt and pepper to taste.

Instructions:

Preheat the oven to 400 °F (200 °C).

Arrange the salmon fillets on a baking pan lined with parchment paper.

Drizzle olive oil over the fillets and season with dill, lemon juice, salt, and pepper.

Bake for 12-15 minutes, or until salmon flakes readily with a fork.

This recipe is tasty and nutritious, making it an excellent choice for any dinner group.

Vegetarian and Vegan Meals

Eating plant-based does not need losing flavor or satisfaction. These vegetarian and vegan recipes are nutritious and delicious.

Stuffed Bell Peppers

Stuffed bell peppers are not only visually stunning, but they also provide a nutritious and satisfying lunch.

Recipe: Quinoa and Black Bean Stuffed Bell Peppers

Ingredients:

4 large bell peppers, half with seeds removed.

1 cup cooked quinoa.

1 can black beans, drained and rinsed.

Eloke

1 cup corn, frozen or canned.

1 teaspoon cumin.

1 teaspoon of chili powder.

Add salt and pepper to taste.

1/2 cup shredded cheese (optional)

Instructions:

Preheat the oven to 375°F (190° C).

In a bowl, combine the quinoa, black beans, corn, cumin, chili powder, salt, and pepper.

Fill the bell pepper halves with the mixture and set in a baking dish.

If using, sprinkle cheese over the stuffed peppers.

Cover with foil and bake for 30 minutes. Remove the foil and bake for another 10 minutes.

These stuffed peppers are full and healthful, making them an excellent supper choice for the entire family.

Creamy vegan pasta

Pasta may be a delicious dinner option, especially when coupled with a dairy-free cream sauce.

Recipe Idea: Creamy Avocado Pasta

Ingredients:

12 ounces pasta of your choice (gluten-free if necessary)

Two ripe avocados.

2 cloves garlic

Juice from 1 lemon

¼ cup fresh basil

Add salt and pepper to taste.

Cherry tomatoes for garnish (optional).

Instructions:

Cook the pasta according to the package instructions. Save ½ cup of spaghetti water before draining.

In a blender, combine the avocados, garlic, lemon juice, basil, salt, and pepper. Blend until smooth.

In a large bowl, combine the cooked pasta and avocado sauce, adding leftover pasta water as needed to get the desired consistency.

Serve with cherry tomatoes if preferred.

This creamy pasta dish is rich, tasty, and can be made in under 30 minutes!

Flavorful Stir-Fry

Stir-fry is a quick and varied dinner choice. They are perfect for using up leftover vegetables and proteins, making them both cost effective and simple to cook.

Chicken and Vegetable Stir-Fry

This colorful and flavorful chicken stir-fry is an excellent dinner choice that can be prepared quickly.

Recipe Idea: Stir-Fry with Chicken and Vegetables

Ingredients:

1 pound chicken breast, thinly sliced

2 tablespoons of soy sauce (verify for fructose-free).

2 tablespoons of vegetable oil.

1 cup snap peas.

1 bell pepper, sliced

One carrot, sliced

2 garlic cloves, minced

Cooked rice for serving.

Instructions:

Marinate the cut chicken in soy sauce for 10 minutes.

Heat 1 tablespoon oil in a pan over medium-high heat. Stir-fry the chicken until cooked through. Remove from the skillet.

In the same skillet, combine the remaining oil, snap peas, bell pepper, carrot, and garlic. Stir-fry until vegetables are soft and crunchy.

Return the chicken to the skillet and stir to incorporate. Serve with cooked rice.

This stir-fry is quick, simple, and ideal for a hectic weeknight.

Tofu and Broccoli Stir-Fry

This tofu stir-fry is a tasty and comforting plant-based alternative that is also high in protein.

Tofu and Broccoli Stir-Fry

Ingredients:

1 block of firm tofu, pressed and cubed

2 cups broccoli florets.

2 tablespoons soy sauce (make sure it is fructose-free)

1 tablespoon of sesame oil.

2 garlic cloves, minced

1 tablespoon cornstarch (optional for crispy tofu)

Optional: To make crispy tofu, coat the cubed tofu in cornstarch before frying.

Heat the sesame oil in a large skillet over medium-high heat. Add the tofu and fry until browned on all sides. Remove and set aside.

In the same skillet, cook the broccoli and garlic for about 5 minutes, or until the broccoli is soft but still vivid.

Return the tofu to the skillet, add the soy sauce, and stir until thoroughly incorporated. Serve with rice or quinoa.

This tofu and broccoli stir-fry is a healthful and satisfying dinner alternative that non-vegans will like!

Dinner may be a pleasurable event even if you follow a fructose-free diet. These recipes allow you to prepare dinners that are both delicious and flavorful. These meals, which include herb-roasted chicken and lemon garlic butter shrimp as well as stuffed bell peppers and creamy vegan pasta, are intended to appeal to a wide range of tastes. Stir-fries provide convenience, allowing you to prepare great dinners quickly.

So grab your ingredients, turn on the burner, and enjoy these Dinner Delights to make every evening memorable. Whether you're cooking for family, friends, or just yourself, each recipe provides an opportunity to try new flavors and appreciate the joy of wonderful cuisine. Happy cooking!

Chapter 5, Snacks and Appetizers

Snacking is an important component of our daily food consumption, and it does not have to be sacrificed when you follow a fructose-free diet. In this chapter, we'll look at delicious and nutritious snacks and appetizers that meet your nutritional demands without sacrificing flavor. Whether you're craving something sweet, savory, or a combination of the two, these recipes will keep you pleased between meals and at gatherings with friends and family.

Nutritious snack bars

Homemade Fructose-free Granola Bars

Store-bought granola bars are frequently loaded with hidden sugars, but preparing your own is not only simple but also gives you complete control over the contents. This recipe combines oats, almonds, and seeds to make a delightful snack that's ideal for on-the-go situations.

Ingredients:

2 cups rolled oats.

1 cup mixed nuts (almonds, walnuts, and pecans).

1/2 cup seeds (pumpkin and sunflower seeds)

1/2 cup unsweetened coconut flakes.

1/2 cup almond butter.

1/4 cup maple or agave syrup.

1/2 teaspoon of vanilla extract.

1/2 teaspoon of cinnamon.

A pinch of salt.

Instructions:

Preheat the oven to 350°F (175° C). Line a baking dish (approximately 9x9 inches) with parchment paper, leaving enough overhang for easy removal.

In a large bowl, combine the oats, mixed nuts, seeds, coconut flakes, and salt.

In a small saucepan over low heat, combine almond butter, maple syrup, vanilla essence, and cinnamon. Stir until melted and smooth.

Pour the wet ingredients into the dry mixture and whisk until thoroughly incorporated.

Press the mixture firmly into the lined baking dish, ensuring even distribution.

Bake for 20-25 minutes, till golden brown. Allow it to cool completely before cutting into bars. Store in an airtight container.

These granola bars are crunchy, filling, and ideal for a midday snack or post-workout treat!

Chocolate-Dipped Nut Clusters

When you're craving something sweet, these chocolate-dipped nut clusters are a quick and guilt-free treat.

Ingredients:

1 cup of mixed nuts (your choice)

1/2 cup dark chocolate chips (make sure they are fructose-free).

Sea salt is optional.

Instructions:

Line a baking sheet with parchment paper.

In a microwave-safe bowl, melt dark chocolate chips in 30-second intervals, stirring after each one until smooth.

Stir the combined nuts into the melted chocolate until thoroughly coated.

Using a spoon, place clusters of the mixture onto the prepared baking sheet.

Sprinkle with sea salt if preferred.

Refrigerate until the chocolate has hardened.

These delicious clusters are ideal for sharing or as a quick sweet treat when cravings strike!

Dip and Spread

Dips and spreads are ideal for parties and casual gatherings. They can be served with a variety of accompaniments, including veggie sticks, low-fructose crackers, or just on their own. The following two dishes are sure to impress a crowd.

Creamy avocado dip.

This avocado dip is rich, creamy, and extremely adaptable. It can be served as a dip for vegetables or spread on your favorite gluten-free toast.

Eloke

Ingredients:

Two ripe avocados.

1 tablespoon of lime juice.

1 clove garlic, minced

Add salt and pepper to taste.

A sprinkle of cumin (optional).

Instructions:

In a mixing basin, mash the avocados with a fork.

Mix in the lime juice, minced garlic, salt, pepper, and cumin, if using.

Serve immediately alongside vegetable sticks or as a spread.

Roasted Red Pepper Hummus.

Traditional hummus frequently includes chickpeas, which may not be suitable for everyone. This roasted red pepper hummus is a flavorful alternative that is ideal for dipping.

Ingredients:

2 large roasted red peppers, jarred or homemade.

1 cup sunflower seeds.

1/4 cup tahini.

2 teaspoons of lemon juice.

1 clove garlic.

Salt to taste.

Add water as needed to achieve consistency.

Instructions:

In a food processor, combine the roasted red peppers, sunflower seeds, tahini, lemon juice, garlic, and salt.

Blend until smooth, then add water one spoonful at a time until the desired consistency is obtained.

Serve alongside low-fructose crackers or vegetable sticks.

These dips are not only nutritious, but also popular at every event, guaranteeing that everyone has something tasty to eat.

Baked Products

Baked products are frequently considered snacks, but they might be difficult to consume on a fructose-free diet. However, with the correct ingredients, you may make delicious sweets that everyone will enjoy.

Coconut Flour Muffins

Coconut flour is an excellent substitute for standard flours, offering a moist texture and delicate sweetness without the fructose. These muffins are ideal as a breakfast or afternoon snack.

Ingredients:

1/2 cup coconut flour.

1/4 cup almond flour.

1/4 cup melted coconut oil.

Three huge eggs.

1/4 cup unsweetened applesauce or pumpkin puree

1/4 cup maple or agave syrup.

1 teaspoon of baking soda.

1/2 teaspoon of vanilla extract.

A pinch of salt.

Instructions:

Preheat the oven to 350°F/175°C and line a muffin tray with liners.

In a mixing basin, combine the coconut flour, almond flour, baking soda, and salt.

In another bowl, combine the eggs, melted coconut oil, applesauce, maple syrup, and vanilla extract.

Mix the wet and dry ingredients until well combined.

Fill each muffin liner with about two-thirds of the batter.

Bake for 20–25 minutes, or until a toothpick inserted in the center comes out clean.

These muffins are light and fluffy, and make an excellent grab-and-go snack!

Savory cheese biscuits.

These savory cheese biscuits are ideal for an appetizer or snack, and will appeal to both children and adults.

Ingredients:

1 cup almond flour.

1/2 cup shredded cheddar cheese (or your preferred cheese)

1/4 cup melted coconut oil.

One huge egg.

1/2 teaspoon of baking powder.

Add salt and pepper to taste.

Instructions:

Preheat the oven to 350°F/175°C and line a baking sheet with parchment paper.

In a mixing dish, combine the almond flour, shredded cheese, baking powder, salt, and pepper.

In another bowl, combine the melted coconut oil and the egg.

Mix together the wet and dry ingredients, stirring until a dough forms.

Scoop tablespoon-sized chunks onto the baking sheet and space them approximately 2 inches apart.

Bake for 15-20 minutes, until golden.

These cheese biscuits are crispy on the outside, soft on the inside, and incredibly tasty!

Quick bites: chips and popcorn.

Crunchy textures are frequently preferred when munching. Chips and popcorn are popular, and with a little creativity, you can make your own fructose-free alternatives that are delicious.

Kale Chips

Kale chips are a healthier alternative to regular potato chips. They're crisp, tasty, and simple to prepare.

Ingredients:

One bunch of washed and dried kale

1 tablespoon of olive oil.

Salt to taste.

Optional flavorings include garlic powder, paprika, or nutritional yeast.

Instructions:

Preheat the oven to 350°F/175°C and line a baking sheet with parchment paper.

Separate the kale leaves from the stems and break them into bite-sized pieces.

Toss the kale in a bowl with the olive oil and salt, being sure to coat each piece.

Spread the kale in an equal layer on the baking sheet.

Bake for 10-15 minutes, until the edges are crisp but not browned.

These kale chips are the ideal guilt-free snack to satisfy your crispy cravings.

Sweet and Savory Popcorn

Popcorn can be a delicious snack, especially when properly seasoned. This recipe allows you to go sweet or savory, depending on your mood.

Ingredients:

1/2 cup of popcorn kernels.

2 tablespoons coconut oil.

Optional ingredients for savory dishes include garlic powder, salt, and nutritional yeast; for sweet dishes, cinnamon, chocolate powder, or maple syrup.

Instructions:

In a large pot, melt the coconut oil over medium heat. Add the popcorn kernels and cover the pot.

Shake the pot occasionally until the popping has subsided to a few seconds between pops.

Once popped, transfer to a big bowl.

Season to taste: mix with savory spices or sweet powders.

Popcorn is a terrific snack that can satisfy both sweet and salty tastes, making it an adaptable addition to your snacking arsenal.

This chapter has featured a variety of snacks and appetizers that are both delicious and suitable for a fructose-free lifestyle. Whether you're craving something sweet, like chocolate-dipped nut clusters, or something savory, like creamy avocado dip, these recipes are intended to satisfy your needs while remaining healthy.

Each recipe is designed to allow you to snack without feeling limited by your dietary restrictions.

Chapter 6: Desserts.

Dessert is one of life's greatest joys, yet people who avoid fructose may feel deprived of sweet sweets. However, with the correct ingredients and a little creativity, you can make delectable treats that will not make you feel terrible. In this chapter, we'll look at a variety of appealing recipes, including cakes and cookies, frozen treats, and fruit-free options. Let's get into the realm of fructose-free desserts that will fulfill your sweet taste!

Fructose-free Sweeteners

Before we get into the recipes, it's important to understand the sweeteners that can be used as sugar alternatives. Many conventional sweeteners are high in fructose, which can be troublesome for people trying to restrict their use. Fortunately, there are various fructose-free sweeteners available that may be used to make delicious desserts without losing flavor.

Options to consider:

Stevia is a natural sweetener obtained from the Stevia plant's leaves. It is a strong sweetener with no calories or fructose. It has far greater sweetening power than sugar, so a little goes a long way.

Erythritol: This sugar alcohol is roughly 70% sweeter than sugar and contains no calories or fructose. It does not cause high blood sugar levels, making it a good alternative for diabetics.

Monk Fruit Sweetener: This sweetener, made from monk fruit extract, is gaining popularity due to its natural ingredients and zero calorie count. It can be used in a 1:1 ratio with sugar.

Allulose: This low-calorie sweetener has the same taste and texture as sugar but has no calories or fructose. It's an excellent choice for baking and cooking.

Xylitol: Another sugar alcohol, xylitol, has a similar sweetness to sugar but should be used with caution around pets because it is poisonous to dogs.

Using these sweeteners, you may make delightful treats that fit your dietary needs and fulfill your sweet tooth.

Cakes & Cookies

Chocolate Chip Cookies.

Who doesn't enjoy a basic chocolate chip cookie? These cookies are thick, chewy, and ideal for fulfilling your sweet tooth.

Ingredients:

1 1/2 cups almond flour.

1/2 cup erythritol or your favorite sweetener.

1/4 cup melted coconut oil.

One huge egg.

1 teaspoon of vanilla extract.

1/2 teaspoon of baking soda.

1/4 teaspoon salt.

1/2 cup of sugar-free chocolate chips.

Instructions:

Preheat the oven to 350°F/175°C and line a baking sheet with parchment paper.

In a mixing dish, combine the almond flour, erythritol, baking soda, and salt.

In another bowl, combine the melted coconut oil, egg, and vanilla essence.

Add the wet components to the dry ingredients gradually, mixing well after each addition.

Fold in the sugar-free chocolate chips.

Place tablespoon-sized bits of dough on the prepared baking sheet, spacing them approximately 2 inches apart.

Bake for 10-12 minutes, until the edges are golden brown.

Allow to cool before enjoying!

These cookies are a certain way to add cheer to any dessert table!

Vanilla Bean Cake.

This luscious vanilla bean cake is ideal for birthdays, parties, or simply because you deserve a treat.

Ingredients:

2 cups almond flour.

1/2 cup erythritol or your favorite sweetener.

1/2 cup unsweetened applesauce.

Eloke

Four big eggs.

1 teaspoon of vanilla extract.

1 tablespoon vanilla bean paste (or seeds from one vanilla pod)

1 teaspoon of baking powder.

1/2 teaspoon of salt.

Instructions:

Preheat the oven to 350°F/175°C and grease a circular cake pan.

In a mixing bowl, whisk together almond flour, erythritol, baking powder, and salt.

In a separate bowl, mix together the applesauce, eggs, vanilla essence, and vanilla bean paste until smooth.

Add the dry ingredients to the liquid components gradually, mixing until well blended.

Pour the batter into the prepared cake pan and level up the top.

Bake for 25–30 minutes, or until a toothpick inserted in the center comes out clean.

Allow to cool before serving.

This cake can be served plain or with your favorite frosting, such as whipped coconut cream.

Frozen treats.

Creamy Coconut Ice Cream.

Ice cream is a popular treat, and this creamy coconut ice cream is a great option that's simple to make and quite tasty.

Ingredients:

2 cans of full-fat coconut milk

1/2 cup erythritol or your favorite sweetener.

1 tablespoon of vanilla extract.

A pinch of salt.

Instructions:

In a mixing dish, add the coconut milk, erythritol, vanilla extract, and salt.

Whisk until the sweetener is completely dissolved.

Pour the ingredients into an ice cream maker and churn according to the manufacturer's directions until it becomes creamy.

Place in an airtight container and freeze for at least two hours before serving.

This coconut ice cream is delightful and ideal for a hot summer day!

Chocolate Avocado Mousse

This chocolate avocado mousse is rich, creamy, and indulgent, and it will surprise and please your friends and family.

Ingredients:

Two ripe avocados.

1/4 cup unsweetened cocoa powder.

1/4 cup erythritol or your favorite sweetener.

1/2 cup almond milk.

1 teaspoon of vanilla extract.

Instructions:

In a food processor, blend the avocados, chocolate powder, erythritol, almond milk, and vanilla extract.

Blend until smooth and creamy, scraping down the sides as necessary.

Taste and adjust the sweetness if necessary.

Spoon into separate serving dishes and chill at least 30 minutes before serving.

This mousse is not only flavorful, but it also contains healthy fats!

Fruit-free delights.

For individuals who want to skip fruits entirely, these dessert recipes can fulfill your sweet tooth without any fruity flavors.

Peanut Butter Chocolate Cups

These peanut butter chocolate cups are a delicious treat that resembles the iconic Reese's cup but lacks the fructose.

Ingredients:

1 cup natural peanut butter, unsweetened

1 cup sugar-free chocolate chips.

1/4 cup erythritol (optional).

Instructions:

Line a muffin tray with cupcake liners.

In a microwave-safe bowl, melt the chocolate chips in 30-second intervals while stirring until smooth.

Pour just enough melted chocolate to coat the bottom of each cupcake liner.

Place the muffin tray in the freezer for approximately 10 minutes to let the chocolate to solidify.

Meanwhile, combine the peanut butter and erythritol until completely blended.

Remove the muffin tray from the freezer and place a spoonful of the peanut butter mixture on top of the chocolate layer.

Pour enough melted chocolate over top to completely cover the peanut butter.

Return to the freezer for an additional 15-20 minutes to set.

These chocolate cupcakes are a delectable treat that will keep you satisfied!

Almond Flour Brownies

Brownies are a classic treat, and these almond flour brownies are decadent, fudgy, and really wonderful.

Ingredients:

1/2 cup almond flour.

1/2 cup unsweetened cocoa powder.

1/4 cup erythritol or your favorite sweetener.

1/4 cup melted coconut oil.

Two huge eggs.

1 teaspoon of vanilla extract.

1/2 teaspoon of baking powder.

A pinch of salt.

Instructions:

Preheat the oven to 350°F/175°C and butter an 8x8-inch baking pan.

In a mixing dish, whisk together almond flour, cocoa powder, erythritol, baking powder, and salt.

In a separate dish, mix together the melted coconut oil, eggs, and vanilla extract until smooth.

Add the wet components to the dry ingredients gradually, mixing until well blended.

Pour the batter into the prepared baking pan and distribute evenly.

Bake for 20 to 25 minutes, or until a toothpick inserted in the center comes out clean.

Let cool before cutting into squares.

These brownies are ideal for a sweet treat after dinner or as a mid-day snack.

Desserts do not have to be avoided just because you are following a fructose-free diet. With the correct ingredients and ingenuity, you may make delectable desserts that everyone will enjoy. From classic cookies to luscious mousses and indulgent frozen delights, these recipes are sure to satisfy your cravings without jeopardizing your diet. So go ahead and treat yourself to something delicious; you deserve it.

Chapter 7: Meal Plan

Consuming a fructose-free diet does not imply abandoning flavor or diversity. With careful planning and preparation, you can enjoy tasty meals that meet your dietary requirements. In this chapter, you will get a one-week fructose-free meal plan, shopping lists, substitutes for popular foods, and helpful recommendations for dining out safely. Let's explore the amazing world of meal planning!

One Week's Fructose-Free Meal Plan

Day 1:

Breakfast: Spinach smoothie with unsweetened almond milk and a scoop of protein powder.

Lunch: Quinoa salad with cucumber, bell peppers, and lemon vinaigrette.

Dinner: Grilled chicken breast with roasted broccoli and sweet potatoes.

Snack: Carrot sticks and hummus.

Day 2:

Breakfast: Chia pudding with coconut milk and sunflower nuts.

Lunch: Lettuce wraps with turkey, avocado, and a drizzle of olive oil.

Dinner: Stir-fried beef with bell peppers and zucchini served over brown rice.

Snack: Rice cakes with almond butter.

Day 3:

Breakfast: oatmeal topped with walnuts and cinnamon.

Lunch: Spinach salad with grilled shrimp, avocado, and balsamic vinaigrette.

Dinner: Baked salmon with asparagus and quinoa.

Snack: Celery sticks with peanut butter.

Day 4:

Breakfast includes scrambled eggs with spinach and feta cheese.

Lunch: Chickpea salad with sliced cucumber, tomatoes, and lemon dressing.

Dinner: Turkey meatballs served with zucchini noodles and marinara sauce.

Snack: almonds.

Day 5:

Breakfast: A smoothie bowl topped with coconut flakes and nuts.

Lunch: Grilled vegetable wrap with hummus on a gluten-free tortilla.

Dinner: Roasted chicken thighs served with Brussels sprouts and carrots.

Snack: Greek yogurt with chia seeds.

Day 6:

Breakfast: Egg muffins made with eggs, cheese, and chopped vegetables.

Lunch: lentil soup with spinach and spices.

Dinner is pork chops with sautéed green beans and cauliflower mash.

Snacks include cheese slices and cucumber rounds.

Day 7:

Breakfast: Pancakes cooked with almond flour served with sugarless syrup.

Lunch consists of zucchini fritters served with mixed greens on the side.

Dinner: Shrimp tacos with lettuce leaves, avocado, and lime dressing.

Snack: Dark chocolate (sugar-free) and a handful of nuts.

This meal plan stresses balanced nutrition while keeping fructose levels low. Feel free to mix and match meals according to your preferences!

Shopping Lists and Substitutions

Making a shopping list is essential for staying organized and ensuring that you have all of the supplies you need to cook your meals. Here is a detailed grocery list based on the one-week meal plan:

Proteins:

Chicken breast

Ground turkey.

Eloke

Beef Strips

Salmon fillets

Shrimp

Eggs

Canned chickpeas

Lentils

Almond butter

Peanut Butter

Grains and legumes:

Quinoa

Brown rice

Gluten-free oats.

Rice cakes

Gluten-free tortillas.

Vegetables:

Spinach

Broccoli

Zucchini

Bell peppers

Sweet potatoes

Cucumbers

Carrots

Celery

Brussels sprouts

Asparagus

Mixed greens

Fruit (low-fructose alternatives):

Avocado

Bananas (in moderation).

Berries: strawberries, blueberries

Dairy and alternatives:

Coconut milk

Unsweetened almond milk.

Greek yogurt (unsweetened).

Cheese (hard variations).

Nuts and seeds:

Almonds

Walnuts

Chia seeds

Sunflower seeds

Coconut flakes

Condiments and spices:

Olive oil

Balsamic vinegar

Lemon juice

Cinnamon

Vanilla extract.

Sugar-free marinara sauce.

Sweeteners:

Erythritol

Stevia

Substitutions:

Choose gluten-free bread or lettuce wraps.

For pasta, use zucchini noodles or spaghetti squash.

If you want a creamy texture, add avocado or tahini instead of dairy.

Check the labels on packaged foods to be sure they're fructose free.

Tips For Dining Out Safely

Eating out while on a fructose-free diet might be difficult, but with the right methods in place, you can enjoy restaurant meals without anxiety.

Restaurant Research: Look for restaurants that have customizable menus or that specialize in fresh, natural foods. Ethnic cuisines such as Mediterranean and Asian frequently offer a variety of options.

Check Menus in Advance: Many restaurants make their menus available online. Reviewing the menu ahead of time will help you select what to order and report any changes to the staff.

Communicate with Your Server: Do not hesitate to inquire about specific ingredients or preparation methods. Tell them about your dietary limitations, and they will most likely be flexible.

Choose Whole Foods: Eat meals that contain whole ingredients, such as grilled meats, steamed veggies, and simple salads. Avoid sauces that may contain hidden sugars.

Substitutions: Request substitutions wherever possible. For example, instead of fries, serve steamed vegetables or a side salad.

Portion Control: Restaurants frequently serve greater portions than are necessary. Consider splitting a dish or saving leftovers for later.

Avoid Buffets: Buffets can be difficult to navigate because the components in each dish are not always obvious. If you go to a buffet, select items that are simple and straightforward.

Stay Hydrated: Choose water or unsweetened beverages over sugary ones. This can help you avoid cravings for sweet foods and stay hydrated.

Dessert: If you want dessert, ask the restaurant if they can make anything special for you or if there are any sugar-free options.

By following these guidelines, you can enjoy dining out without jeopardizing your dietary requirements.

Meal preparation may be a fun activity, especially when it comes to preparing delicious, fructose-free dishes. You may maintain a healthy lifestyle while indulging in satisfying meals by following a well-structured meal plan, creating a careful shopping list, and understanding how to handle dining out. Enjoy cooking and trying new flavors while keeping your fructose intake under control. Happy eating!

Chapter 8: Helpful Resources

Navigating a fructose-free lifestyle can be difficult, but with the appropriate materials at your disposal, you can empower yourself to make informed decisions, stay inspired, and connect with others who are on the same path. This chapter includes a complete list of safe foods, useful resources for further reading, and online groups where you can seek help and share your experiences. Let's look at some useful tools to assist you live a fructose-free life.

List of Safe Foods

Knowing which foods are safe to eat when living a fructose-free lifestyle is critical for keeping a balanced diet. The following is a curated list of fructose-free food options divided into different categories:

Proteins

Fresh cuts of chicken, turkey, cattle, lamb, hog, and fish (avoid processed meats containing high-fructose corn syrup).

Eggs are a flexible protein source that may be prepared in different ways.

Dairy products include hard cheeses (cheddar and Swiss), plain Greek yogurt (unsweetened), and dairy or lactose-free milk.

Legumes: Lentils, chickpeas, and most beans (black, pinto, kidney) in moderation.

Grains

Gluten-free options include rice, quinoa, oatmeal, and cornmeal.

Bread: Gluten-free bread and tortillas (avoid additional sweeteners).

Gluten-free pasta prepared with rice or quinoa.

Fruits (low fructose)

Berries: Eat strawberries, blueberries, and raspberries in moderation.

Citrus: lemons, limes, and oranges (in moderation).

Other options include bananas, cantaloupe, and honeydew melon (with moderation).

Vegetables

Leafy greens include spinach, kale, and lettuce.

Root vegetables include potatoes, carrots, and sweet potatoes.

Cruciferous vegetables include broccoli, cauliflower, and Brussels sprouts.

Other vegetables include zucchini, bell peppers, cucumbers, and green beans.

Nuts and seeds.

Nuts include almonds, walnuts, pecans, and macadamia nuts.

Chia seeds, flaxseeds, and sunflower seeds.

Oils and Fats

Healthy oils include olive, coconut, and avocado oil.

Butter: When cooking and baking, use unsalted butter or ghee.

Sweeteners

Fructose-free sweeteners include erythritol, stevia, and monk fruit sweetener.

Homemade Alternatives: While unsweetened applesauce can be consumed in moderation, it should be taken with caution due to its fructose concentration.

These healthy food selections will assist you in developing a variety and fulfilling diet while limiting your fructose consumption. Remember to read the labels on packaged items, as many include hidden sugars and high-fructose corn syrup.

Conclusion

Embracing a fructose-free lifestyle demands courage, perseverance, and adaptability. After exploring the various facets of this lifestyle throughout the book, you now have a toolkit of knowledge, recipes, and support tools to assist you traverse this route with confidence. As we end up, let's talk about encouragement and practical ideas for sticking to this lifestyle, as well as some closing thoughts on health and nutrition.

Encouragement & Tips for Leading a Fructose-Free Life

Embrace the Journey: Transitioning to a fructose-free diet may appear difficult at first, but remember that each step toward greater health is a success. Celebrate your accomplishments, no matter how modest, and be nice to yourself amid failures. The journey is equally vital as the destination.

Continue Learning: Maintain your curiosity about food and nutrition. Inform yourself on the most recent research on fructose intolerance and its treatment. This will allow you to make more educated choices and change your diet as needed. Knowledge is your greatest ally!

Plan Ahead: Meal planning is an effective technique for sticking to your fructose-free lifestyle. Set up time each week to plan your meals and snacks. Having a well-stocked kitchen with safe foods reduces the temptation to go for harmful options when hunger strikes.

Experiment in the Kitchen: Use this occasion to try out new dishes and ingredients. Cooking should be enjoyable and imaginative. Experiment with new flavors, textures, and cuisines that are compatible with your fructose-free diet. This can make meals more engaging and reduce boredom.

Listen to Your Body: Notice how different foods make you feel. Everyone's tolerance levels vary, so pay attention to your body's responses. If required, keep a food diary and record everything you consume as well as any symptoms you have. This practice might help you detect patterns and improve your diet.

Connect with Others: Do not be afraid to reach out to friends, family, and online communities. Sharing your experiences, struggles, and accomplishments can help to build a supporting network, making the journey less isolated. You'll discover that many people can connect and are eager to provide advice and encouragement.

Focus on Whole Foods: Base your diet on whole, unadulterated foods that are naturally low in sugar. These foods not only support a fructose-free lifestyle, but they also improve general health. To make balanced meals, add plenty of veggies, whole grains, lean proteins, and healthy fats.

Stay Hydrated: Water is crucial for overall health, especially while switching up your diet. Drink plenty of drinks throughout the day to stay hydrated. Herbal teas and infused water with healthy fruits can bring diversity and taste to your hydration routine.

Seek Professional Help: If you're having trouble or your symptoms aren't improving, talk to a certified dietitian or nutritionist who specializes in food intolerance. They can offer personalized guidance and support to help you manage your diet properly.

Be Patient: Transitioning to a fructose-free lifestyle does not happen overnight. It takes time to adapt, locate appropriate alternatives, and form new habits. Be patient with yourself, and realize that progress happens gradually.

Final thoughts on health and nutrition

As you wrap up this voyage into the world of fructose intolerance, it's critical to consider the broader implications of health and nutrition in your life. Nutrition is more than just what you eat; it includes your total well-being, mental health, and lifestyle choices. Adopting a fructose-free diet can be a catalyst for good transformation, resulting in a healthier relationship with food and a higher quality of life.

Prioritize Balanced nutrients: Eating fructose-free does not imply abandoning nutrients. Include a variety of nutritious foods in your diet. Aim for balance, ensuring that you are getting enough vitamins, minerals, and macronutrients to maintain good health.

Cultivate Mindful Eating: Practice mindfulness in your eating habits. Slow down, taste each bite, and heed to your body's hunger and fullness signals. This practice can improve your connection with food by allowing you to appreciate the flavors and experiences associated with each meal.

Invest in Your Health: View your health as a lifetime investment. Make mindful decisions that promote your physical and mental well. This includes emphasizing regular physical activity, stress management, and adequate sleep, all of which are critical to your overall health.

Advocate for Yourself: As you learn more about fructose intolerance, don't be afraid to advocate for yourself in social situations or while dining out. Clearly explain your dietary requirements and preferences to friends, family, and restaurant workers. Your health is worth advocating for!

Adopt a Holistic Approach: Remember that health is multifaceted. Along with nutritional modifications, think about other components of wellbeing, such mental health, emotional well-being, and physical activity. Meditation, yoga, and writing can all help you stay on track with your nutrition and promote overall wellness.

Stay Inspired: Keep the flame of inspiration alive by exploring new recipes, cooking techniques, and cuisine trends. Follow food bloggers, take cooking classes, or attend workshops about healthy eating. The more involved you are, the more fun your journey will be.

Reflect on Your trip: Take regular time to reflect on your trip and progress. Recognize your progress and enjoy your successes. This self-reflection can strengthen your resolve and determination to live a fructose-free lifestyle.

Be adaptable: While it is critical to follow a fructose-free diet, life is about balance. Allow yourself to indulge occasionally without feeling guilty. It's great to indulge yourself on occasion; what matters is how you respond and then resume your good routines.

Finally, adopting a fructose-free lifestyle entails more than just avoiding certain foods; it also entails taking a comprehensive approach to health and nutrition. As you continue down this path, remember that you have the ability to make choices that improve your well-being, bring joy to your meals, and connect with a supportive community. Your trip is unique, and with determination and the correct resources, you can complete it successfully.

Thank you for joining me on this journey through fructose intolerance and the delectable benefits of a fructose-free diet. May you find joy in every meal, strength in your decisions, and health on your journey.

Here's to a vibrant, fructose-free future!

Thank You for Reading!

I want to take a moment to personally thank you for choosing to read fructose-free living. Your time and effort are sincerely appreciated, and I hope this book has provided you with significant ideas and skills for success.

As I continue to grow as an author, your feedback is immensely essential to me. I would love to hear your thoughts—whether positive or constructive—so I can grow and make future works even more helpful and fascinating.

If you found this book beneficial or if there's something you feel could be enhanced, I respectfully ask that you provide an honest review. Your insights will not only help me improve but also assist other readers in locating the correct information.

Thank you again for your support, and I look forward to hearing from you!

Warm regards,

The end

Made in the USA
Las Vegas, NV
27 December 2024

15468621R00075